The Narcissist Next Door

Simple steps on how to recognize and Manage Toxic Relationships

Paul J. Edwards

Copyrights© Paul Edwards

All rights reserved. No part of this book may be used or reproduced in any form whatsoever without written permission form the author or her publishers except in the case of brief quotations in critical articles or reviews.

TABLE OF CONTENTS

INTRODUCTION

CHAPTER ONE
Decoding the Narcissist

CHAPTER TWO
The Masks They Wear

CHAPTER THREE
Emotional Puppetry

CHAPTER FOUR
The Cost of Deception

CHAPTER FIVE
Drawing the Line

CHAPTER SIX
The Turning Point

CHAPTER SEVEN
The Art of Disengagement

CHAPTER EIGHT
Reclaiming Your Self

CHAPTER NINE
The Empowered Ally

CHAPTER TEN

Beyond the Shadow
NOTES

THIS PAGE IS INTENTIONALLY LEFT BLANK

INTRODUCTION

In every community, workplace, and social setting, a hidden threat lurks that can disrupt relationships and impact lives: the narcissist. These individuals, often charismatic and persuasive, have a way of captivating those around them while masking their true, more harmful nature. **"The Narcissist Next Door: Recognizing and Managing Toxic Relationships"** aims to shed light on the hidden dangers posed by these personalities and equip you with the strategies needed to navigate and reclaim your personal space from their toxic influence.

Understanding Narcissism:

At its essence, narcissism is marked by an excessive focus on oneself, coupled with a notable absence of empathy and a relentless need for admiration. Narcissists are skilled at manipulating perceptions and presenting a façade that hides their genuine nature. This book provides a foundation for grasping how narcissists operate, their impact on others, and why they present such significant challenges in both personal and professional spheres.

Why This Book Is Important:

Dealing with narcissists can be exceptionally difficult. Their manipulative tendencies often leave others feeling confused, invalidated, and isolated. By elucidating the nature of narcissistic behavior, this book aims to empower readers to identify these individuals, understand their tactics, and develop effective methods for managing their influence.

Many people unknowingly find themselves in toxic relationships with narcissists, struggling to understand why these interactions are so draining and harmful. This book offers clarity, serving as a guide for those currently dealing with such relationships and as a preventive resource for recognizing early warning signs and avoiding potential pitfalls.

What You Will Learn:

The Narcissist Next Door explores various facets of narcissistic behavior and its impact on relationships. Each chapter is designed to enhance your understanding, from recognizing narcissistic traits to applying practical strategies for managing interactions and reclaiming your well-being.

Identifying Traits: Discover both subtle and overt signs of narcissism to help you determine whether someone in your life exhibits these characteristics.

Understanding Dynamics: Gain insight into the psychological mechanisms behind narcissistic behavior and its effects on relationships.

Practical Strategies: Learn actionable techniques for managing interactions with narcissists, including setting boundaries, safeguarding your emotional health, and seeking support when needed.

Empowerment and Recovery: Follow the guidance on healing and rebuilding your sense of self after encountering toxic relationships.

The Journey Ahead

Managing relationships with narcissists demands patience, self-awareness, and resilience. This book serves as a comprehensive guide, combining psychological insights with practical advice. As you begin this journey, remember that recognizing and addressing narcissistic behavior is not just about handling difficult interactions—it's about reclaiming your life and surrounding yourself with supportive, healthy connections.

Welcome to **"The Narcissist Next Door."** Here, you will find the knowledge and tools necessary to confront and overcome the challenges presented by narcissistic individuals, setting the stage for healthier, more fulfilling relationships and a stronger, empowered self.

CHAPTER ONE

Decoding the Narcissist

Unraveling the Complexities of Narcissistic Behavior

Understanding the many facets of narcissism can be difficult, especially if you find yourself entangled in its web. It is crucial to understand the complex nature of narcissistic behavior before attempting to deal with a narcissist. By exploring the psychology of narcissism, this chapter clarifies the motivations for and expressions of these actions.

Why Narcissism Is Psychological

Narcissism Definition:

Narcissism is clinically defined by an inflated sense of self-importance, an intense craving for admiration, and a lack of empathy towards others. According to the DSM-5, narcissistic personality disorder (NPD) is marked by a persistent pattern of grandiosity, a strong need for admiration, and an absence of empathy.

Psychological Foundation: Narcissism can develop due to a combination of early life experiences and genetic factors. Various conditions, such as childhood trauma, excessive pampering, and overpraise, can contribute to the emergence of narcissistic traits.

Different Narcissistic Personalities:
Overt narcissism is typified by overt conceit, a need for praise, and an overt show of superiority. Grandiose behavior and a self-centered mindset make overt narcissists easy to spot.
Contrarily, *covert narcissists* manipulate their targets more subtly. They may appear shy or sympathetic, yet they lack empathy and have a strong need for approval. Even if their actions are less overt, they can still be harmful.

Expression in Various Personas:

Leaders Who Exude Charm: Those who are overtly narcissistic frequently project a pleasant and captivating demeanor, which positions them as apparent leaders. Although their boldness and confidence can at first draw attention, they gradually display a deeper, more dangerous drive for control.

Martyrs Who Have Been Victimized: Narcissists in disguise may pose as victims or martyrs to appeal to others' compassion and manipulate them by appearing weak. This facade conceals their fundamental desire for approval and dominance

Recognizing the Narcissistic Features

Magnificence and Personal Worth:

Exaggerated Sense of Self: Narcissists frequently believe they are better than others and should be given preference.
This conceit might show itself as a
persistent craving for adulation, boasting, and bragging.
Entitlement: Narcissists feel they are entitled to a particular treatment and may become irate or resentful if their demands are not fulfilled.

Emotional Disconnect: Narcissists have trouble understanding the feelings and experiences of other people. They largely prioritize their own wants and needs, which causes them to be indifferent to the needs and sentiments of people around them.

Manipulative Behavior: Narcissists can take advantage of people by manipulating them, frequently with no regrets or regard for the emotional toll they take on their victims. This is made possible by their lack of empathy.

Manipulation and Management:

Psychological Manipulation Techniques:

Narcissists use a range of manipulation techniques, including gaslighting, in order to stay in charge and evade responsibility. The victim's sense of self may be damaged by these strategies, which can warp reality.

CHAPTER TWO

The Masks They Wear

Recognizing the Facades of Narcissism

Narcissists are adept at wearing different masks to manipulate and control others while concealing their true selves. This chapter explores the various personas narcissists project and how these facades are used to manipulate others and achieve their goals.

The Charmer's Mask

Entertaining Persona:

First Impressions: Narcissists frequently project a pleasant, charismatic image that captivates people with their assurance and charm. An first impression of likeability and magnetism may be produced by this charm.
Manipulative Intent: A manipulative intent is concealed beneath the charm. The narcissist uses charm as a tactic to win others over, earn their

trust, and create openings for more manipulation.

Creating Trust:

First Attraction: Narcissists can appear sincere and reliable due to their charisma. To establish a good rapport, they could show interest, flattery, and acts of compassion.
Once trust has been built, the narcissist may start to subtly manage and manipulate, utilizing their original appeal as a tool.

The Martyr's Mask of the Victim

Taking on the Role of the Victim:

Perceived Vulnerability: To gain sympathy and control over others, covert narcissists frequently dress themselves as martyrs who have suffered greatly. To inspire sympathy and support, they would present themselves as downtrodden or misunderstood. To increase the likelihood that someone will submit to the narcissist's demands or ignore their destructive behavior, this mask is utilized to instill guilt in others.

Bending the Emotional Heart:

Narcissists take advantage of others' pity and compassion by portraying themselves as victims. To avoid taking responsibility for their acts and to divert criticism, they put on this mask.
Using the victimized martyr's mask, a narcissist can exert control over others by influencing their thoughts and feelings.

The Majestic Leader's Mask

Giving Off Confidence:

Authority: Narcissists may exhibit confidence and authority by donning a grandiose leader's mask. In order to bolster their sense of superiority, they would assume leadership responsibilities and pursue positions of authority.
Demanding Respect: This character is frequently paired with requests for adoration and respect, which serves to bolster the narcissist's sense of entitlement and superiority.

Making Use of Power:

Authoritarian Control: The narcissist uses the guise of the grandiose leader to impose control and power over others. Their sense of dominance and power may be strengthened by their use of manipulation, intimidation, and dominance.

The Unconfident Mask

Assessing Suitability:

False humility: In an attempt to get comfort and approval from others, narcissists may put on an insecure mask and project vulnerability or self-doubt.

Self-Deprecation: This façade may entail remarks or actions that are meant to make one feel better about oneself and get support.
Tricking the Senses:

Seeking validation: Narcissists can coerce people into giving them continual affirmation and comfort by wearing an insecure facade. It also acts as a way for them to escape accountability for their actions.

CHAPTER THREE

Emotional Puppetry

Understanding Narcissistic Manipulation Tactics

Master manipulators and narcissists use a variety of strategies to subjugate and take advantage of their victims. This chapter examines the several strategies employed by narcissists to manipulate people in relationships, such as psychological games, manipulation, and emotional blackmail.

Psychological Coercion

The meaning and workings:

Idea: Emotional blackmail is the practice of forcing someone to comply by instilling feelings of duty, guilt, or fear. Emotional blackmail is a tactic used by narcissists to keep control and get their way.
strategies: Using guilt trips, playing on the victim's fears, or threatening to withhold

affection are common strategies.

Examples and Their Significance

Examples from Personal Experiences: A narcissistic spouse may use the fear of abandonment as a coercive method to get what they want out of the relationship.
Emotional Repercussions: The victim of emotional blackmail may experience anxiousness, insecurity, and a helpless feeling.

Gaslighting

The meaning and workings of:

The idea behind gaslighting is to manipulate someone's perceptions of reality and themselves using psychological tricks. Gaslighting is a tactic used by narcissists to confuse and cause doubt in their victim.

Methods: Methods consist of forcing the victim to doubt their sanity and memory, fabricating information, and rejecting prior experiences.
Examples and Their Significance

Individual Cases: An employee may begin to doubt their memory if their narcissistic employer, for instance, insists on not acknowledging that they clearly recall a directive.

Emotional Consequences: Gaslighting can cause profound emotional discomfort, such as bewilderment, self-doubt, and a weakened sense of reality.

Taking on the Victim Persona

Definition and Workings:

Idea: In order to win others over, escape accountability, and control them, narcissists frequently adopt a victim role. They can deflect responsibility and garner support by using this strategy.
Exaggerating one's own struggles, presenting oneself as the victim, and attempting to win over too much sympathy are examples of tactics.
Case Studies and Their Effects:

Personal Examples: To get attention and avoid

accepting accountability for their actions, a narcissistic buddy could exaggerate their problems.

Implications for Emotions: A vicious cycle of codependency and enabling can result from playing the victim, in which the victim is continuously attempting to please or save the narcissist.

Triangulation

Definition and Mechanisms:

Concept: Triangulation involves introducing a third party into a conflict to create division and manipulate dynamics. Narcissists use triangulation to control relationships and incite jealousy or competition.

Techniques: Techniques include comparing the victim to others, creating conflict between individuals, and using third parties to manipulate the victim's emotions.

Examples and Impact:

Personal Examples: For example, a narcissistic parent might compare their child to a more successful sibling to foster rivalry and control behavior.

Emotional Consequences: Triangulation can lead to feelings of inadequacy, jealousy, and strained relationships with others.

CHAPTER FOUR

The Cost of Deception

Emotional Fallout from Narcissistic Relationships

Narcissistic relationships can inflict deep emotional wounds, significantly harming self-esteem, mental health, and overall well-being. This chapter explores the emotional and psychological toll of enduring relationships with narcissistic individuals over time.

Diminished Self-Worth

Impact on Self-Esteem:

Relentless Criticism: Victims of narcissists often endure ongoing belittlement and criticism, which gradually erodes their self-esteem. This constant negativity wears down their sense of personal value.

Developing Self-Doubt: The repeated negative remarks and critiques from a narcissist can lead victims to question their worth and abilities.

Restoring Self-Worth:

Rebuilding Confidence: Recovery involves challenging and changing the negative beliefs implanted by the narcissist. Utilizing positive self-talk and setting achievable goals can help in regaining self-esteem.

Restoring a Positive Self-Image: Self-compassion and recognizing one's strengths are essential in reconstructing a healthy self-image.

Mental Health Struggles

Depression and Anxiety: Prolonged exposure to narcissistic behavior can lead to emotional instability, manifesting as anxiety, depression, and a sense of hopelessness.

Seeking Therapy: Professional counseling and the development of coping strategies are vital for addressing these mental health challenges.

Trauma Indicators:

Post-Traumatic Stress Disorder (PTSD): Some individuals may suffer from symptoms like recurring nightmares, flashbacks, and heightened vigilance as a result of their trauma.

Healing from Trauma: Overcoming these symptoms requires professional support and self-care practices that nurture mental health and well-being.

Enduring Effects of Manipulation

Trust Issues:

Difficulty Trusting Others: Experiencing manipulation and deception can make it challenging to trust others in future relationships. Overcoming these fears is often a significant hurdle for survivors.

Building Trust Gradually: Establishing healthy, trusting relationships involves gradually learning to trust those who are truly reliable.

Fear of Repeating Negative Patterns:

Avoiding Toxic Relationships: Individuals who have experienced narcissistic abuse may fear slipping back into destructive patterns in other relationships. Setting firm boundaries and learning from past experiences are crucial in preventing a recurrence.

Promoting Self-Awareness and Growth: Through self-awareness and personal development, individuals can identify and avoid falling into harmful relationship dynamics.

CHAPTER FIVE

Drawing the Line

Establishing Boundaries with Narcissists

Setting and maintaining boundaries with narcissists is crucial for safeguarding yourself from further harm and preserving your emotional independence. This chapter outlines strategies for effectively establishing boundaries and asserting your personal space.

Understanding Boundaries

Definition and Importance:

What Are Boundaries: Boundaries are the limits or guidelines that define acceptable behavior and protect an individual's well-being. They are vital for maintaining healthy relationships and ensuring emotional safety.

Purpose of Boundaries: Boundaries help shield you from manipulation, assert your personal needs, and prevent others from overstepping.

Types of Boundaries:

Physical Boundaries: These pertain to personal space and physical interactions. It's essential to communicate and enforce your limits on physical contact and proximity.

Emotional Boundaries: These involve protecting your emotional well-being by limiting exposure to manipulation and ensuring your feelings are respected.

Setting Boundaries with Narcissists

Clear Communication:

Defining Limits: Clearly state your boundaries and expectations to the narcissist. Be explicit about what behaviors are unacceptable and what you require to feel respected and safe.

Maintaining Consistency: Enforce your boundaries consistently to emphasize their importance and prevent the narcissist from testing or crossing them.

Assertiveness:

Assertive Behavior: Use assertive communication to express your needs and limits confidently, without aggression or hesitation. Use "I" statements to convey how specific behaviors impact you.

Handling Pushback: Be prepared for resistance or attempts to undermine your boundaries. Stay firm and consistent in upholding your limits.

Protecting Emotional Autonomy

Avoiding Emotional Manipulation:

Recognizing Manipulation: Be aware of the tactics narcissists use to manipulate your emotions and perceptions. Identify when you are being subjected to emotional blackmail or gaslighting.

Maintaining Emotional Distance: Practice emotional detachment to protect your well-being. Focus on your feelings and needs rather than getting entangled in the narcissist's manipulations.

Prioritizing Self-Care:

Self-Care Practices: Engage in activities that support your emotional and physical health. Prioritize what brings you joy, relaxation, and fulfillment.

Building Support Networks: Surround yourself with supportive people who respect your boundaries and offer positive reinforcement.

CHAPTER SIX

The Turning Point

Deciding When Enough is Enough

A crucial decision in managing toxic relationships is figuring out when to confront, separate from, or break off contact with a narcissist. How to identify the tipping moment and make wise decisions are covered in this chapter.

How to Determine the Tipping Point

Alerts for an Escalation:

Growing Toxicology: Keep an eye out for indicators that the level of toxicity in the relationship is rising, such as emotional abuse, more frequent manipulation, or a worsening of mental health issues.

Diminishment of Health: Take notice of any changes in your personal health, such as increased anxiety, depression, or low self-esteem. The connection may be getting more damaging based on these indicators.

Concerns for Emotion and Pragmatics:

The relationship's emotional impact on your general well-being and emotional condition should be considered.

Ask yourself if staying in the relationship will be more beneficial emotionally or not.

Realistic Elements: Evaluate realistic factors, like how it will affect your everyday obligations, aspirations, and life in general. Think about your long-term health and whether continuing the relationship makes sense.

Picking a Side to Face or Leave

A confrontation

When to Face It: If you think facing it would help the relationship work out or become better, then go ahead and do it. Strive to communicate your needs during the talk by making clear, concise remarks.

In managing A confrontation You should be ready for the narcissist to deny or resist. While keeping emotional clarity and control, be assertive and firm.

Betweenness and Distancing:

Gradual Detachment: Evaluate progressively removing yourself from the narcissist if confronting them is neither practical nor productive. Minimize communication and establish physical and emotional space.

Emotional distance: To safeguard your wellbeing, concentrate on maintaining emotional distance. Take care of yourself and partake in activities that strengthen your sense of autonomy and self-worth.
severing bonds

Forming the Choice:

Assessing Necessity: Choose if severing links is the best course of action for your health. Think about if you need to be apart for your health or if the relationship is too damaged to repair.
Arranging for Disturbance: Make arrangements for the practical and psychological difficulties that may come up while severing ties. If you need assistance, ask dependable people or experts.

Putting the Separation into Practice:

Effective Communication: Make sure to express your decision in a forceful and clear manner. Establish limits for upcoming communications and make sure your choice is acknowledged.

Post-Separation Support: To overcome any practical or emotional obstacles, get help both during and after the separation process. To aid in your recuperation, take up healing and self-care activities.

CHAPTER SEVEN

The Art of Disengagement

Techniques for Emotionally Detaching from a Narcissist

Emotionally detaching from a narcissist is vital for regaining control over your life and ensuring your emotional safety. This chapter delves into strategies for disengaging emotionally, limiting interactions, and prioritizing self-preservation.

Limiting Contact

Reducing Interaction:

Practical Measures: Gradually decrease the amount and duration of contact with the narcissist. This may include setting boundaries around communication methods and reducing in-person encounters.

Avoiding Provocations: Recognize and steer clear of topics or scenarios that are likely to provoke conflicts or manipulative behavior.

Upholding Boundaries:

Consistent Application: Enforce your boundaries consistently to prevent the narcissist from encroaching upon your limits. It's crucial to remain firm in maintaining the distance necessary for your well-being.

Managing Attempts at Reconnection: Be prepared for the narcissist to attempt to re-enter your life or challenge your boundaries. Stay committed to your goal of reducing contact.

Reframing the Relationship

Changing Your Perspective:

Altering Perceptions: Reassess your view of the relationship, acknowledging its unhealthy and manipulative nature. Dismiss any lingering idealizations or false hopes you may have had.

Focusing on Reality: Keep your attention on the true impact of the narcissist's behavior on your mental and emotional health. Resist getting caught up in their distorted views or attempts to twist reality.

Adopting an Emotionally Detached Approach:

Maintaining Emotional Distance: Practice emotional detachment to diminish the influence of the narcissist's behavior on your feelings. This involves mentally and emotionally distancing yourself from their manipulative actions.

Prioritizing Self-Care: Focus on self-care and activities that reinforce your sense of self-worth and independence. Engage in practices that support your emotional strength and recovery.

Focusing on Self-Preservation

Rebuilding Your Identity:

Rediscovering Self-Worth: Engage in activities and build relationships that strengthen your sense of self-worth and identity. Place emphasis on personal growth and self-awareness.

Setting New Goals: Define new personal and professional aspirations that align with your values and desires. Use this time to explore interests and passions that bring you fulfillment.

Strengthening Resilience:

Developing Coping Mechanisms: Develop strategies to manage any lingering effects of the narcissistic relationship. This may involve practicing mindfulness, seeking therapy, or participating in support groups.

Building a Support Network: Surround yourself with supportive individuals who respect your boundaries and contribute positively to your life.

CHAPTER EIGHT

Reclaiming Your Self

Rediscovering Your Identity After Narcissistic Influence

Healing from a relationship with a narcissist requires a deep reconnection with your authentic self and a dedicated effort to rebuild your sense of worth. This chapter delves into the process of self-recovery, highlighting the importance of reclaiming your values, restoring your self-esteem, and pursuing a life that is meaningful and fulfilling.

Reconnecting with Core Values

Reflecting on Personal Principles:

Understanding Your Core Beliefs: Take time to reflect on the core beliefs and values that may have been suppressed or overlooked during the narcissistic relationship. Identify what is truly important to you and what defines your unique identity.

Aligning Life with Your Values: Begin to make decisions and take actions that align with your true values. Engage in activities and relationships that honor and support these principles.

Rediscovering What Brings Joy:

Re-engaging in Enjoyable Activities: Reconnect with hobbies and passions that once brought you joy or explore new interests that resonate with your true self. These activities can help restore your sense of identity and provide a source of fulfillment.

Building Confidence Through Pursuits: Participate in activities that reinforce your self-confidence and self-esteem. Celebrate the small successes and progress you make as you reclaim your sense of self.

Restoring Self-Esteem

Addressing Negative Self-Perception:

Challenging Harmful Thoughts: Identify and counteract any negative beliefs or self-talk that may have been ingrained by the narcissist. Replace these thoughts with positive affirmations and practice self-compassion.

Recognizing Your Strengths: Focus on acknowledging and appreciating your strengths and achievements. Celebrate your resilience and the unique qualities that make you who you are.

Embracing Positive Reinforcement:

Incorporating Daily Affirmations: Use positive affirmations daily to reinforce your sense of self-worth and confidence. Choose affirmations that affirm your value and encourage self-love.

Visualizing a Positive Self-Image: Practice visualization techniques to imagine a future where you feel empowered and successful. Picture yourself achieving your goals and living in alignment with your true values.

Crafting a Life That Reflects Your True Self

Setting and Achieving Personal Goals:

Establishing Meaningful Objectives: Set personal and professional goals that reflect your core values and aspirations. Develop a clear plan to achieve these goals and take consistent steps toward them.

Pursuing Growth and Development: Actively seek opportunities for personal growth and self-improvement. Embrace challenges that contribute to your development and help you learn more about yourself.

Fostering Healthy Connections:

Building a Supportive Network: Surround yourself with people who respect and support your identity. Cultivate relationships that are positive and uplifting, and that respect your boundaries.

Maintaining Healthy Boundaries: Continue to establish and enforce boundaries in all areas of your life. This is crucial for protecting your emotional well-being and ensuring that your relationships remain healthy and supportive.

CHAPTER NINE

The Empowered Ally

Supporting Others Trapped in Narcissistic Dynamics

Supporting loved ones who are entangled with a narcissist demands a careful approach that blends empathy with actionable advice. This chapter offers insights into how to assist them while respecting their independence and encouraging their empowerment.

Offering Emotional Support

Listening with Compassion:

Providing a Non-Judgmental Space: Create a supportive and non-judgmental environment where your loved one can openly share their feelings and experiences. Listen actively and show understanding, validating the challenges they face without dismissing their emotions.

Acknowledging Their Struggles: Recognize and affirm the emotions and experiences they're going through, offering them reassurance and empathy. Make sure they know you're there for them without pushing them to make immediate decisions.

Sharing Practical Advice:

Providing Useful Resources: Offer them information about narcissistic behavior and the dynamics of healthy relationships. Suggest they explore therapy, support groups, or relevant self-help materials to aid their journey.

Encouraging Self-Care: Encourage them to focus on self-care, engaging in activities that support their physical and emotional health. Suggest practices like mindfulness, exercise, or journaling to help them manage their well-being.

Empowering Their Decision-Making

Respecting Their Autonomy:

Avoiding Pressure: Empower them to make decisions on their own terms without applying pressure or coercion. Support their choices, ensuring they align with their personal values and contribute to their overall well-being.

Supporting Their Process: Be there to guide and encourage them, but allow them to take the lead in their decision-making. Offer your support without taking control of the situation.

Promoting Healthy Boundaries:

Discussing the Role of Boundaries: Explain the importance of setting and maintaining clear boundaries with the narcissist. Offer advice on how to establish these boundaries effectively and protect their emotional health.

Reinforcing Self-Empowerment: Encourage them to recognize their strengths and to take proactive steps toward safeguarding their well-being. Highlight their resilience and support their journey toward self-empowerment.

Avoiding Enabling Behaviors

Recognizing Enabling Patterns:

Identifying Enabling Behaviors: Be aware of actions that may inadvertently enable the narcissist, such as excusing their behavior or downplaying its impact. Help your loved one recognize and avoid these patterns.

Encouraging Firm Boundaries: Support them in setting and maintaining strong boundaries with the narcissist, ensuring they don't become enmeshed in manipulative tactics.

Fostering Positive Change:

Promoting Growth and Healing: Encourage them to make positive changes in their life and relationships. Support their pursuit of professional help, goal-setting, and personal growth as they move forward.

CHAPTER TEN

Beyond the Shadow

Thriving in a Life Free from Narcissistic Influence

Emerging from a narcissistic relationship marks the beginning of a transformative journey towards personal growth, the formation of healthy connections, and a deeper sense of empowerment. This chapter offers insights and strategies for thriving after such a relationship, focusing on personal development and creating a fulfilling future.

Pursuing Personal Development

Rediscovering Interests:

Reconnecting with Passions: Set aside time to rediscover activities and interests that you enjoyed before the relationship. Engaging in these pursuits can reignite your sense of joy and fulfillment.

Defining New Goals: Establish fresh personal and professional goals that align with your true values. View this period as an opportunity for self-discovery and growth.

Strengthening Emotional Resilience:

Cultivating Inner Strength: Build emotional resilience through self-care, mindfulness practices, and affirmations. Enhance your ability to manage and overcome life's challenges.

Gleaning Lessons: Reflect on the lessons learned from the relationship and use these insights to foster growth and improve future interactions.

Fostering Healthy Relationships

Building Positive Connections:

Creating Supportive Environments: Surround yourself with trustworthy and supportive individuals. Seek relationships based on mutual respect and genuine understanding.

Maintaining Boundaries: Establish and enforce boundaries to ensure your relationships are balanced and respectful. Guard against falling into unhealthy patterns.

Engaging in Meaningful Interactions:

Forming Authentic Relationships: Pursue interactions that align with your personal values and interests. Build connections that contribute to your well-being and personal growth.

Making Positive Contributions: Offer support and kindness to others, using your experiences to contribute positively to your community and relationships.

Crafting a Fulfilling Life

Exploring New Opportunities:

Embracing New Experiences: Be open to exploring new opportunities that resonate with your goals and values. Engage in activities that bring satisfaction and joy.

Vision for the Future: Develop a clear vision for your future that reflects your aspirations. Take proactive steps to build a life that aligns with your authentic self.

Practicing Self-Compassion:

Prioritizing Self-Care: Engage in regular self-care to support your physical and emotional well-being. Foster a positive self-relationship through compassion and self-kindness.

Celebrating Achievements: Recognize and celebrate your progress and accomplishments. Acknowledge your strength and resilience in moving past previous challenges.

NOTES

www.ingramcontent.com/pod-product-compliance
Lightning Source LLC
Chambersburg PA
CBHW070418230526
45471CB00006B/2868